M000042914

NPH:

Journey into Dementia and Out Again

By Sharon French Harris with Hugh Harris

Second Edition

Sharon French Harris with Hugh Harris

ISBN: 978-1549610820

WORDQUILT BOOKS
North Chesterfield, Virginia

Dedication

To family, friends, pray-ers, and medical providers who have seen me through this journey.

□□□

NPH is often an insidious disease which is difficult to diagnose, but as in the case of Ms. Harris, when diagnosed and treated, a life can truly be changed. The first time I saw Mrs. Harris after her surgery, the change in her was remarkable. She was back to the woman I had known for years. Her story had a very happy ending and every time I see her, I smile. I am grateful she shared her story.

--Caroline P. Cella, M.D.

Sharon French Harris with Hugh Harris

Table of Contents

Introduction

Normal Pressure Hydrocephalus (NPH): An abnormal accumulation of cerebrospinal fluid in the ventricles (cavities) of the brain.

"The normal path of development through our adult lives includes fairly stable periods followed by periods of internal turmoil and transition. During these times, we take another look at who we are, how we relate to others, and what we want to do with our lives. These stages give us the chance to grow, but they carry the risk of decline as well. Our success or failure in dealing with these transitions determines how well we move on through the important phases of our lives." Morford, Hungar and Willing in Life After 60? Yes!

Unveiling

By Hugh Harris

What happened? It seems only minutes since I left you sitting on that bench under the light, while I ran back to retrieve my forgotten cap. There—in the distance—is that—you? Bent over, shuffling steps, pocketbook dragging the ground. No, it's some old woman, lost, in a fog. So vulnerable.

I go closer. It is you. I call, "Sharon?" You answer, "I can't find the car." So, it begins on a dismal night in Williamsburg, the gradual recession into a world of lost gait, tumbled balance, trembling hands, blocked memory, unruly bladder. What day is it? What year? What time? What's your name? Who is the President? Touch your nose. Recall this string of words. Benchmarked tests, yearly repeats, "Mild Cognitive Impairment." Up at night—can't sleep. Falling down the stairs. Falling in the garage. Falling through the veil of reality into a hidden realm of confusion.

"You have drop foot." "Get a brace." It helps—but not for long. Enter placard-guaranteed parking; next a chair on wheels. So many obstacles, steps, doors that don't open automatically. Incontinence relief. "Depends" in constant supply. Where's the bathroom? Change the meds. Continence improves, urge still rages. Words formed in thought, jumbled in verbalization. Disorientation: What day is it? What's the use? Where are we going? Have you seen Hugh? Who's going to get me up today? When can we go home?

New tests. Mild cognitive impairment significantly advanced. Normal Pressure Hydrocephalus? Scans show enlarged ventricle. Excessive cerebrospinal fluid no longer absorbed, impacts brain function. A sliver of hope. Claim it. Pray for it and believe your own prayers. Another fall brings daily trained care at home. Surgery scheduled. Do a spinal tap, see what symptoms are relieved. The door back to reality cracks open. Go through it, boldly.

Surrounding voices cry, Caution. Maybe it won't work. Don't get your hopes up. Silence. Hope that doesn't anticipate isn't hope. It's delusion. We have hope. Report for neurosurgery Monday morning. Thanks be to God.

Preface

"The dead man came out, his hands and feet bound with strips of cloth, and his face wrapped in a cloth. Jesus said to them, 'Unbind him, and let him go.'" (John 11:44 NRSV)

No one could have been more surprised than I when I went for my first annual gynecological examination at age 19. The doctor palpated my neck and said, "I believe you have a thyroid gland that is malfunctioning. I'm going to refer you to an endocrinologist for further tests and study."

After seeking a second opinion which confirmed the gynecologist's suspicion, I had a partial thyroidectomy. When I ordered a copy of the pathology report, it stated there were several benign nodules. The remainder of my thyroid gland was removed when I was 60 years old due to what turned out to the development of more benign nodules. Before surgery this time, however, my doctor handed me a computer disc to take home after my visit. When I saw the size and number of the nodules, I decided the removal of the rest of my thyroid gland had been a good decision.

My purpose here is to tell about my experience with Normal Pressure Hydrocephalus. I mention hypothyroidism because it, like depression from which I also suffer, has many symptoms in common with NPH. All three share symptoms of fatigue, decreased energy, disturbance in sleep pattern, and difficulty with concentration, detail retention and decision making. With each there are complaints of aches or pains, headaches, some concern about going out in public, and disinterest in formerly pleasurable activities.

The result can be withdrawal from many daily activities. These symptomatic similarities can make it difficult to determine exactly what is happening. Hopefully, by sharing my journey, I can contribute to the body of knowledge about NPH and its effects, as well as give hope and encouragement to people who suffer from such symptoms.

Over the last few years I have found myself on a wild and at times unfathomable ride. I fell into a nightmare that affected all dimensions of my life—mental, physical, emotional, psychological, spiritual and relational. I experienced an improbable journey into dementia at a far-too-early age. By the grace of God, I was surrounded by caring people of faith who held hope before me. Now I have returned, unbound from the debilitating symptoms that had wrapped my life in shrouds of confusion and uncertainty.

In the pages that follow, I have asked my husband Hugh to share the unfolding of this journey with me, because he made the trip as my life's companion, patient advocate, and caregiver. We will each share our perspective on what was happening at various stages of the journey.

Among the many people who have seen me through this journey is my sister-in-law, who raised the question more than four years ago about whether I might have NPH. I felt relieved to have a name I could attach to what I was experiencing, but I soon found that dealing with what the name represented was an intricate matter that took time.

She had read in the Sunday newspaper supplement, *Parade Magazine,* about an athlete who was diagnosed with NPH after suffering from a concussion. That seemed to make everything I had experienced in cognitive decline fall into place. I will tell you about a fall where I hit my head on my car, denting it no less, and then fell onto the garage's cement floor. Looking back, I wonder if that blow could have caused NPH?

My first CT Scan showed only minimal abnormalities that might have been connected to a concussion. I wasn't that old yet (just 61), and I knew incontinence was a sign of aging. Hadn't Florence Henderson been in Depends commercials on television for years? Without some unifying clarification, these things just didn't add up. The medical diagnosis NPH provided that clarification, but much of my journey revolved around verifying NPH as a valid diagnosis, and then wrapping my condition around it to produce healing.

—Sharon

ooo

On January 1, 1999, my eighty-six-year-old father died at the skill care facility where he had spent his closing years with Alzheimer's Disease (AD). He had lived most of his last decade with this gradually deepening condition that stole his personality. I still remember his withdrawal, apprehension, anger, and conversation that was unrelated to the present. With each passing month, he receded farther back into things that had happened in his young adulthood, youth and then childhood. AD didn't take him away with a sudden sweeping blow but slowly swallowed him into a private world from which he could not be extricated and into which his family could not go.

When Sharon experienced cognitive decline, there was some rumbling in the background about the possibility that she was descending into irreversible dementia. Some of her symptoms seemed to suggest AD, Parkinson's Disease (PD), or Traumatic Brain Injury (TBI), but both of us always knew there was a difference. We were familiar with AD through my dad's experience, and her uncle had PD for nearly three decades.

Sharon gradually developed a bilateral tremor in her hands that worsened over time. Her short-term memory began to decline noticeably, and her unsteady gait created increasing falls. In fact, she took eight sessions of physical therapy for balance and gait issues. She wore a leg brace that was prescribed by a physical therapist. It helped for a while. Next Sharon began to experience debilitating incontinence. In addition, she would often stare absently when I spoke to her, making no visible or audible response.

Unlike my dad's AD, Sharon's experience was like an express train hurtling through some tunnel we couldn't yet define. Dad took years to traverse this decline, but with Sharon I sometimes felt as if I was seeing measurable changes daily. Somewhere within myself I knew this was all going too fast. When my sister-in-law flagged the possibility of NPH, I looked it up online, and then asked doctors if this might apply to Sharon. Neurological tests did not indicate anything definitive, although the possibility of NPH surfaced early in neuropsychological tests, and was kept alive in the background.

Finally, there came a time when enough pieces came together that Sharon was tested for NPH with a spinal tap and 72-hour observation period. Disappointingly, her responses did not conform to the medical protocol. Then some things changed so that a ventricular-peritoneal shunt was implanted in her brain, and she began her remarkable return trip from dementia to normal cognitive functioning. Hers was a recovery of a miraculous dimension, worth sharing with others to give hope and encouragement.

We have written this together, combining her skills as a former English teacher and Licensed Professional Counselor and Marriage and Family Therapist, with mine as a pastor and writer. Every day is a celebration of Sharon's return from symptoms so typical of dementia that at one point she did not even know who I was. We are each sharing our own recollections at each stage, mine first as her caregiver, followed by her perceptions until the point when her cognitive functioning had become so normal that she speaks for herself.

Throughout this journey we were each aware of God's presence with us, and our faith sustained us with a certainty that all things were happening within God's time. Our prayer is that you will find his blessings in your own journey, and that our experience will be helpful to many people throughout the world.

—Hugh

1
Early Warnings

Hugh

It was a brisk March evening when Sharon and I entered the Kings Arms Tavern in historic Williamsburg, Virginia, to celebrate our mutual birthday. We share a somewhat unique circumstance of having been born on the same day of the same month, although eleven years apart. The trip to this historic village had become our annual tradition.

Seated at a window table in an upstairs room, we looked down on the street where tourists, groups of school children, and characters in colonial garb paraded by. A horse-drawn carriage passed outside as the server brought our order, and a troubadour began to serenade the room full of diners. All of that was normal, yet I had a sense of dis-ease. Sharon was sitting across from me, yet she seemed distant with a vacant expression in her eyes. I took it as a sign of her fatigue.

After supper, we left the tavern and walked up Duke of Gloucester Street to where we could cut across to the parking area. Darkness had fallen and a damp chill filled the air. We paused amidst a crowd under a street lamp.

"Honey, I need to go back and get my cap. I left it in the tavern." She looked at me with a blank expression. Spying a bench nearby I said, "Why don't you sit here while I run back. I'll only be a few minutes."

She sat down and I sprinted back, picked up the cap and quickly returned. Sharon was nowhere in sight. The bench was vacant. I called out, "Sharon?" No answer. I moved among the crowd asking if anyone had seen where she had gone. No one had noticed her. I began to feel apprehensive and decided to walk toward the parking area. That's when I saw someone under another street lamp, walking feebly, hunched over, almost dragging her purse.

"Sharon?"

No response.

I moved closer. The figure appeared to be that of an elderly woman. *How strange*, I thought. *I wonder if this woman is lost?* Then something in her movement struck me. It *was* Sharon.

"Honey, what's going on? I thought you were going to wait for me."

"Hugh? Where have you been? I've been looking all over for the car."

I reminded her that I'd gone back for my cap and left her on the bench under the light. She didn't recall that. I took her arm and we began walking toward the parking area. I could tell she was cold and tired, and she was quiet as we drove home. It hadn't been a huge incident, yet there was something very unsettling about it.

This occurred just months after I had closed my business as an artist, which I had pursued for eleven years following my retirement from full-time ministry in the United Methodist Church. The business closure was related to the recession and resulted in stressful financial adjustments. Sharon, an English teacher in her first career, was now a Licensed Professional Counselor, and Marriage and Family Therapist, in private practice through a Christian agency where she had worked for nearly fourteen years.

In addition to closing the art business, we also faced the end of a part-time pastorate I had served for five years. Loss of income loomed over us and I have often wondered to what degree the stress of that contributed to Sharon's condition.

The Williamsburg incident was not the first sign of trouble we had seen. On another occasion Sharon had been talking as we drove along a highway near our home. Suddenly her words became jumbled, making no sense. We looked at each other and she stopped talking.

"What did you say?" I asked. "I didn't understand you."

There was a fleeting look of fear in her eyes and she started to say something, but then stopped and sat silently while we drove on another half-mile.

"I don't know what happened," she said. "I couldn't make my words come out right."

Our first thought was that she may have had a mini-stroke. Her mother had experienced several of those over the years, but they had never interfered with her functioning until later in her life. Sharon asked her doctor about it. Tests were made, but there was no evidence of a stroke. We filed the experience away in our minds as perhaps a warning of some sort.

On several occasions in the months prior to, and following, the Williamsburg incident Sharon had experienced disorientation while driving. One time she became confused while on her way to have lunch with her sister-in-law. She called me on her cell phone. "I'm lost. I need for you to come help me find my way out of here. I can't remember the streets." I got her to give me some landmarks so I could find where she was parked. When I got there, she explained that she felt disoriented, so I had her follow me and we drove home without further trouble.

A similar thing happened once when she was to make a presentation in a community north of Richmond off I-95. She had gotten lost trying to find her way from our house to the interstate. When I found her, she was in the parking lot of a senior living complex.

When we finally arrived at our destination, Sharon discovered that someone had stepped in and begun the presentation in her place. We drove back to get her car only to find that the battery was dead. Sharon had forgotten that she'd turned her lights on earlier, and I hadn't noticed it when I picked her up.

Some warnings happened at home. One afternoon when I was sitting in the great room reading, Sharon went into the kitchen to prepare supper. A short time later she called to me. "Can you help me?" I went into the kitchen to see her standing in front of the stove with some utensils out on the counter and a confused expression. Again, her eyes spoke volumes. She said, "I can't remember how to cook." She looked totally defeated.

"Don't worry about it," I said. "We'll do it together." We did manage to get supper on the table, and from then on, I began to do more cooking as her self-confidence in the kitchen seemed to be diminished.

Then there were the falls, which came both before and after the Williamsburg incident. I recall how embarrassed she was once when she came home from work and said she had fallen in the presence of a client in her office. She had tried to stand up, but her feet felt as though they were glued to the floor, so she had fallen in place.

Another time we had just returned from an out-of-town trip and we were each putting things away. I came downstairs to find her upset. "I fell down the garage steps," she said. She had tried to put something on a shelf in the garage, lost her balance, and fallen three steps down to the concrete floor.

I couldn't imagine how she had done that. "Show me what happened."

"I don't know," she replied. "I reached over the railing to put something on the utility shelf and I fell." She rubbed her head and said it hurt. "I bumped my head against the car."

I could see a dent in the left rear quarter panel, but she seemed to have no serious injuries that we could determine. Neither of us thought to take her to the emergency room to be examined. Several other falls occurred during this time. We lived in a two-story Victorian transitional home with carpeted stairs three feet inside the front door. There was a hand railing on the left side of the stairway. The floor at the base of the stairs was linoleum over plywood subflooring.

One day I was in another part of the house when I heard a loud crash coming from the front. Sharon cried out and I rushed in the direction of her voice. I found her lying on her back at the foot of the stairs with her head against the wall beside the front door. She was conscious, but not making much sense.

I called 911, and the paramedics did various tests when they arrived. Because she had no broken bones and no indication of bruises or concussion, they gave us some guidance for avoiding falls. One thing they suggested was installing another railing on the other side of the stairs, which we did. Sharon didn't fall on the stairs after that.

Memory issues also began to occur. I have always had a hard time remembering names and, as a former secondary school and adult learning teacher, Sharon was good at it. For years I relied on her when I would forget a name. Suddenly she lost that skill. Her short-term memory became impaired so that she frequently couldn't remember recent conversations, or what day it was, or what we had on our agenda.

We are people of faith who believe God is with us in all circumstances. Sometimes we can be stubborn and not listen to the obvious. Each of these things that happened—the disorientation at Williamsburg, the temporary aphasia, getting lost while driving over familiar streets, and the falls— all were, we believe, God's *warning signs*. "Listen up," God's Spirit was saying. "Pay attention."

It took a while, but we did get the message.

□□□

Sharon

What I remember most about that night in Williamsburg is how cold it was, and how uncomfortable I felt. I've never been able to endure coldness or dampness easily. I do remember Hugh telling me to sit on the bench while he ran back to get something, and I remember drawing my lined raincoat around me tightly. I think my discomfort overruled all other realities in that moment.

Hugh talks about the stresses related to his loss of the art business and termination of his part-time pastoral position. I remember that those things happened, but I don't recall them as being any more stressful than life in general. I had felt stress about our finances since his retirement in 1999, and his subsequent decision to go into his art as a full-time venture. I have always appreciated his fine artistic talent in several media—it was one of the things that attracted me to him when we first met.

The trouble was that Hugh never seemed able to make much money through art. think I viewed him as a Don Quixote character, riding forth full-tilt with his sword drawn, but with nothing really coming from his efforts. The problem was that there was never a "pay day," a time when the bills were all paid and there was actually money in the bank. There were some times when things went a little better, yet it always felt to me like he was off on a "lark."

This situation had caused periodic friction between us, but I'm not sure what, if any, role that played in my mental health. I think I have understood creative personalities better since being married to Hugh. He has always needed a place, space and time to do his creative work.

Having said that, I do remember clearly the time I went into the kitchen to scramble some eggs. I had cracked them in the bowl. Then my mind went completely blank. I couldn't remember what to do next, and I remember calling him to help me. I think when he took over I just went into the great room and sat down.

I also remember the fall in the garage. We had come back from a trip and I had tried to throw a small insulated bag by its cloth strap across my chest onto a shelf beside the steps. Somehow, I lost my balance. I fell striking my head against the left quarter panel before hitting the concrete floor where I lay for a period of time, calling Hugh for help. I never lost consciousness.

He was upstairs and could not hear me, so I managed to get up and went into the kitchen as he came downstairs. He was alarmed, but since I hadn't passed out and seemed to be recovering, we didn't seek medical help. The back of my head had never hurt as bad. Actually, I was worried as much about the dent in the car as I was about something like head trauma—which I believe now *had happened*.

There were other falls, some of which Hugh didn't mention. Once I fell backwards down the stairs between the first and second floor of the house. I think I tripped over my bedroom slippers as I came down the steps. I somehow twisted my body and landed on my back. Hugh wisely didn't try to move me but called the paramedics who put me in a nearby kitchen chair and checked me out. I was able to tell them accurately the year, month, my name, who the president was—all the questions paramedics use to assess coherence. They didn't feel it was necessary to transport me to the hospital.

Another time we were walking from the mall parking lot toward the entrance to Sears. I didn't perceive the height of the curb and tripped onto a concrete walkway outside the store entrance. That fall produced an abrasion on the palm of my hand where I had tried to catch myself. We put a band aid on that. My hand healed quickly but I felt embarrassed and wondered how I had fallen again for some time afterward.

Then there was my fall on the brick outdoor staircase up to the second-floor entrance to my workplace. I had parked my car and begun climbing the stairs when my feet somehow became tangled and I fell up the stairs, splitting my upper lip. The office manager took me to a Patient First where my wound was treated. I did not need stitches. I never fell on those steps again. Looking back, I remember feeling confused and puzzled by the falls, but I was not fearful.

One of the triad of clinical symptoms for Normal Pressure Hydrocephalus (NPH) is gait disturbance, along with urinary incontinence, and cognitive decline. These incidents clearly show that was happening. My gait was slowing and I was beginning to lean to the left. I remember during worship on Sunday I leaned to the left so severely that I was on a twenty-degree angle to the pew. There were also times when I leaned to the left severely while Hugh was driving our small car. He had to push me to an upright sitting position, even though I was still belted.

Walking felt increasingly laborious and I wanted to avoid it as much as possible. I would have Hugh drop me at the door to a building. He would then go park the car. When we were leaving I would have him bring the car to me at the exit. Even though I don't recall leaning forward and stooping when I walked around looking for the car that night in Williamsburg, I believe Hugh's report is accurate, and I believe I did gradually fall more deeply into that pattern.

NPH has to do with the behavior of a clear cerebrospinal fluid (CSF) that surrounds the brain and spinal cord. The fluid circulates around the brain to deliver nutrients and remove waste products. When extra fluid is produced, the ventricles that produce and store CSF become enlarged, and the fluid may spill out to be absorbed by brain tissue. If too much CSF is present it can cause pressure against different parts of the brain, causing a variety of noticeable symptoms.

Besides the gait issues we've been discussing, it can also affect memory, the ability to reason and solve problems, and speech. In other words, it produces symptoms of what we call *dementia*. In addition, it can create urinary incontinence. The interference with memory can resemble symptoms of Alzheimer's disease, and the gait disturbance can resemble symptoms of Parkinson's disease, so it's easy to misinterpret what's happening. We will be talking more about the symptoms I experienced in the pages ahead.

2

Hills and Valleys

Hugh

As I was staining the deck on a late May afternoon in 2010, I was interrupted by a phone call from the superintendent of the Farmville United Methodist District. "I understand you're looking for a part-time pastoral appointment," he said. "I'm looking for a part-time pastor for the South Halifax Charge, and I wonder if we might be able to work something out that would help us both?"

"Yes, I am looking for something, but that sounds like it would be too far away."

We talked about the details—two small rural churches in the South Boston, Virginia area that was once prime tobacco-producing land that had suffered because of the region's economic decline. We would live in the parsonage on weekends so Sharon could work during the early part of the week. The next day I went with the superintendent to look things over and meet some of the church leaders, and the next day Sharon went with me to see the situation. By the end of the week we had agreed to do it.

At the end of June, we began our weekly, two-hour, 115-mile trek back and forth to Halifax County. During the summer and early fall, there was a relaxed peacefulness that fed my spirit, but Sharon experienced isolation and uprootedness that soon brought on depression in the winter. Sometimes she stayed in Richmond, and I made the trip alone.

Something we hadn't considered also played a role—I was always traveling to hospitals in places like Danville and Lynchburg, Virginia, and Durham North Carolina. Sickness, accidents, funerals and other pastoral needs didn't just happen on weekends. They required travel from Richmond many other days of the week. By the end of our one-year interim pastorate we were glad to return to a life of stability—or so we hoped.

In reality, we returned to the same warning signs that we'd been struggling with before our move to Halifax. We had, in fact, been dealing with them all along. In June 2010, at her request,

Sharon had been referred by her primary care physician to the Memory and Aging Center at the University of Virginia Hospital's neurology department in Charlottesville, Virginia. She was given a diagnosis of Mild Cognitive Impairment (MCI), which was explained as a possible precursor to other forms of cognitive decline, including dementia.

Many of the falls and other situations we have mentioned occurred during this year of traveling back and forth between communities. In the spring of 2011 Sharon had more neurological tests, and consulted again in Charlottesville with the same diagnostic result. We both prayed a lot about these issues, and I remember feeling an inner prodding to make some bold steps as we finished at Halifax.

We had been wanting to sell our two-story house, but the declining housing climate kept deflating the market. During many of our weekends away the house had been shown, but after a few months with no results, we had taken it off the market. "I think we need to try again," I said to Sharon. "How do you feel about that?"

"I agree that we need to try," she said, but we both knew it would be hard to do. Extreme foundation problems had caused us to borrow against the disappearing equity. Finally, we were able to get a sale and to finance the shortfall.

Even before the sale, I had another idea in answer to my prayers. "Why don't we look into the Retired Clergy Housing Corporation (RCHC)?" I asked Sharon, and she agreed. RCHC is an agency of the Virginia Conference that provides retirement housing on a sliding fee for pastors who have spent most of their ministry living in parsonages. We submitted an application and found we qualified. Within weeks RCHC had purchased a house for us and we moved in on October 6. Two days later our house sold.

Now I could see a light at the end of the tunnel, but Sharon couldn't. She fell into a deep depression and some of her cognitive issues began to increase at the same time. She seemed to withdraw into herself so that it was necessary for her to retire from her counseling profession in January 2012. From my perspective, we had been traveling over hills and through valleys for years. God was blessing us with a new tableland in which to dwell with his blessing through a new stage in our lives. Unfortunately, Sharon was not able to share that sense of blessing and hope in the same way that I experienced it.

□□□

Sharon

I simply could not believe that we were going to serve a two-point circuit in Southside Virginia. My practice had suffered as the result of one of the worst recessions the United States had ever known. The inheritance from my parents, which I had invested in mutual funds and an annuity for my retirement, was gone. I felt desperate. I knew I wanted to accompany Hugh on this "adventure," as he called it.

There were some positives. I had always taken Fridays off, and I didn't have enough clients on Thursdays to merit staying home. We would be going to an area of Virginia that I had never seen. I felt that getting away from the trauma I listened to during the week could be helpful. I had a cell phone and a laptop, so my clients and clinical director could reach me in an emergency. It would mean a lot of travel back and forth, but we could do it.

The parishioners would have liked someone to live there full-time, but they understood our circumstances and were accepting toward us. We shared that I had some health problems, but we didn't go into detail about my memory or gait issues. Unfortunately, a medication I had been taking for anxiety and depression had been changed, causing some serious side effects.

One of those was imbalance, and another was auditory hallucinations. There were times when I thought I was losing my mind. All of this helped cloud the neurological issues that were also going on. It would take time to uncover hidden aspects of what I was experiencing.

As I look back, the best part about commuting to Halifax County that year was getting to know some wonderful people at Harmony Church. This was a small church with an average attendance of a dozen people, usually all women, who had deep roots in both their community and their faith. They were loving, accepting people with whom I formed a close bond that year. Their courage and faith in staying with their church in the face of severe economic and social change gave me inspiration for my own struggles.

Hugh speaks of my having been referred to the Aging and Memory Center at UVA, and I'll have to say that for me, it felt like a blessing. I have very positive memories of my visits there. We would walk down the hall while a neurologist observed me and engaged in a routine session of psychological testing at a desk with a computer. I was conscious of being there as a patient, of course, but on the other hand I was also there at a level of academic curiosity. An acquaintance in one of the communities where I had practiced came to mind, and I thought, *Oh, so this is what she did.* Psychological testing always carried an air of mystery, and I wanted to get the best results I could.

When I read the diagnosis of MCI in the report, I felt relief. I was aware of the similarity between my symptoms and those of Alzheimer's and Parkinson's diseases, but I had never felt comfortable with those connections. Now someone was verifying that my instincts had been right. *Good,* I thought, *this is the correct diagnosis.* It helped me feel settled, and I was able to continue my practice and my driving. Looking back, I believe that, while I felt validated by my diagnosis, at the same time, I felt that there was a lot yet to be discovered.

Hugh talks about selling our house and moving into a deed-restricted, 55+ community, and I know the stress of doing that hit me at several points. Even if I hadn't been dealing with a neurological condition, this was a move that would have been hard to take.

For one thing, it was necessitated by circumstances I couldn't control. It also brought the word "aging" to mind. It felt like something that was out-of-place—happening much too soon. In 2008, we had visited the Grand Canyon, where we stood on the rim and looked down at the Colorado River a mile below. Sometimes my life felt as though I was about to go "over the edge," and it was frightening.

Selling our house was a cliff-hanging experience for me. Even though we were selling due to circumstances beyond my control, like falling down the stairs, it still felt to me like I had failed at home ownership. *I should have been able to handle this,* I told myself. After years of living in parsonages owned by the church and maintained by a committee, my spirits had soared when we finally bought our own home as we moved toward retirement.

I had fallen in love with our house the first time I drove past it. I loved the Victorian transitional architecture, the landscaping, the wooded lot, the deck on the back of the house where the terrain dropped away toward a creek. It felt like what my mother-in-law called a "treehouse" when she visited. Across nearly fourteen years we had put our own mark on the house—installed a trendy stone-tile floor in the kitchen, painted all the rooms, wallpapered the bathrooms and kitchen, and in some cases added a new flair by changing furniture.

There was also a down side. We had struggled with constant deterioration of hard board siding, windows that needed replacement, a plumbing problem that had caused us to re-do two bathrooms, and a foundation problem that had caused a corner of the house to sink over two inches, requiring expensive repairs. Somehow the house always seemed to be a "work-in-progress," so leaving it felt like giving up.

Even worse was the feeling of separation from a wonderful next-door neighbor and her husband and children. We had been through two hurricanes and several snow storms together and it hurt to put a dent in the bond we'd formed. At the same time, we only moved a few miles away, so we could maintain our friendship—and we have.

On balance, I was aware that we were being blessed with very good housing through the auspices of the denomination we had served. We were selling a twenty-year-old frame home and moving into an eight-year-old brick home in a gated community. At first, I felt self-conscious about the "gated" part—as though such communities were for people in a socio-economic bracket beyond us. Sometimes I felt like an "imposter." It turned out not to be like that at all.

Our new neighbors were all in the 55+ age bracket, and all were ordinary folks who had a desire for safety and community. We quickly felt blessed to be among them. For the first year or more, however, I felt disconnected from familiarity and had no sense of taking root in our house. I was not in a state of being where I could assimilate change and blossom afresh. It would take time.

During the process of moving, I had felt like a *robot*—going unfeelingly through empty motions. I have tried to find words to describe what I felt. It wasn't despair, which suggests hopelessness to me. It was more like a deep, soul-wrenching disappointment. We were safe, and I settled in, but it just didn't feel like "home."

Looking back, I wonder what role this all played in my cognitive decline. I have decided it was all part of the landscape, but not necessarily causative. I adopted an approach to life where I tried to do what my doctors instructed, taking one day at a time, with a sense of trusting God somewhere in the background of everything.

Developing that attitude made me compliant as a patient, and probably had a lot to do with my being where I am today. t was one of those things where I would say, "Thank God for the experience, and thank God it's over."

3

Uncertain Terrain

Hugh

As we entered 2012 it seemed like Sharon fell into deep depression about having retired from her counseling practice. She became easily confused and struggled with motivation. We tried to keep up with our usual routines. She attended her church circle meetings and we participated in mid-week church suppers, went shopping at the outlet shops in Williamsburg, and dined out with couple friends.

Late in January Sharon wanted to attend a healing service at a local Episcopal church. We had gone there a few times the previous fall, so we returned. She received prayer at the altar. Sharon continued to see her psychiatrist and psychotherapist to deal with depression issues.

The month went along, but without a sense of enthusiasm.

This became the pattern through the spring. We kept up with activities related to the church season, family occasions, and daily routines, but each event seemed more of a struggle for Sharon. Incontinence intensified, and we made adjustments. We had gotten involved with the Lifelong Learning Institute (LLI) by this time and I was involved in an Aspiring Writer's Critique group, while Sharon participated in a French class. She signed up for a second French class, but it had become too much of a challenge for her and she had to back away.

In May Sharon returned for another appointment at the Aging and Memory center in Charlottesville, with the same results. She had MCI. They saw no changes. At the same time, we *felt* changes were happening, even though we couldn't elaborate about them. Doctor visits increased: primary care physician, allergist, psychiatrist, dermatologist, hearing specialist, cardiologist.

During one routine visit to her cardiologist Sharon experienced Atrial Fibrillation. She was sent immediately to the emergency room, where she was admitted for a procedure to correct her sinus rhythm. This was successful and after several days in the hospital she returned home. Now we added in regular visits to a Coumadin clinic to have her International Normalized Ratio (INR) values measured as a precaution against a stroke.

In September, I had an opportunity to attend the 53rd Reunion of the 319th Station Hospital where I had served with the U.S. Army in France. Sharon stayed with a friend for three days while I drove to Ohio and back. When I returned our friend said Sharon had many accidents trying to reach the bathroom, and much difficulty with loss of balance.

We had planned to take a brief trip to the beach at Nags Head, North Carolina, but had to cancel that. I began to see Sharon's condition more realistically, and in October her doctor referred her to a brief rehab program at a local rehabilitation clinic. They diagnosed her balance and walking problems as the result of a drop foot condition, recommending a leg brace and several weeks of rehab exercises, plus home exercises. None of these things really corrected the problem.

An MRI in October showed no change in the enlarged ventricle in her brain. In November, she and I attended a "Keeping the Muse Alive" class at LLI. The classes involved doing creative writing around simple, everyday themes. Sharon couldn't function with this spontaneously, which was noticeable, given her background of teaching secondary school English and journalism (before she retrained and became a counselor).

We would sit down at the dining room table and do our home exercises together. Sharon could pull up some of the images that were called for, but she couldn't remember how to write them with coherence. I learned to talk out her stories with her and then write them in the computer. We would print them out and she would read them in class. This gave her self-esteem a boost.

Back in August we had faced the difficulty Sharon was having walking from the car to stores when we went shopping, so we had gotten a handicapped parking placard through the Division of Motor Vehicles. That enabled us to park closer to store entrances, but we soon found that handicapped parking spaces were often already filled when we arrived. In November, her walking and falling were severe enough that we bought a transport chair, which enabled her to be wheeled around safely in public places. We did not use it at home in the beginning. She had also been using a cane for some time, but her physical therapists had told us it was basically ineffective.

At Christmas, we made a two-day trip to the Shenandoah Valley, staying overnight in a handicapped accessible room at a local hotel. There was a large family gathering for a meal at the facility where my mother lives. Sharon seemed disengaged from family interactions. The trip was a learning experience for what it would take to travel with her growing level of disability. By the end of the year we had a clear sense that things were going downhill with increasing rapidity.

Winter has always been difficult for Sharon. Ice, snow, wind and cold temperatures wear on her spirits in the best of times, and as her disabilities increased, winter became even more of a burden. She ended 2012 with many doctor's appointments that required travel in the cold, so as much as possible beyond that we tried to stay indoors. We felt blessed to have a well-built brick home with a good heating system. All of this, however, increased Sharon's tendency toward depression.

Life felt as if we were traveling over a difficult, always-changing, uncertain terrain, and we both felt off-balance. We prayed together for healing and direction. In my spirit I heard God saying, "Wait. All will be well." It was a hard answer to hear, and I learned to touch base with my spiritual source again each day. That's not to say I was always patient. Sometimes Sharon's lethargy would annoy me. I was increasingly doing more and more to keep her going. I remembered my mother caring for my brother who had Cerebral Palsy. Images of her faith, and times when I remembered her overcoming her own struggles with caregiving, flowed through my mind. Many times I thanked God that I had grown up with her example.

Finally, the year that had become more trying each day, ended. On New Year's evening of 2013, as we had done for many years, Sharon and I sat on the couch together, listening to Johann Strauss compositions performed by the Vienna Philharmonic Orchestra. For a brief moment, we felt a touch of normalcy on the cusp of a new year.

□□□

Sharon

When Hugh began to manage my medications, I was so relieved. That was one less responsibility I had to crowd into my thinking.

I am thankful for the friend of ours who sheltered me while Hugh took a three-day respite trip to his Army veteran's reunion in Marion, Ohio. However, I was mortified when I got up to go to the bathroom and became lost in her house

Concerning my physical therapy for a misdiagnosed drop foot condition, the leg brace did give me some stability, and the therapy sessions did help me have some inner body awareness, but my therapist missed my NPH because I didn't have outward signs other than an "off balance" gait and unsteadiness and reports of falls that weren't severe.

Some of the worst depressions in my life have come between October and May. I have never been diagnosed with Season Affect Disorder (SAD), but I have often wondered if, in addition to my diagnoses of major depressive episodes I may have SAD. My depressive episodes are often related to my sensitivity to loss. Before the onset of each episode over my lifetime I had suffered a great loss.

Hugh did everything he could to normalize life for me. While I don't remember our ritual of watching the New Year's special in 2013, I do remember how he cooked, cleaned, did laundry, and managed everything for us in a time of great uncertainty.

I really believe prayer sustained me during this period of struggle. I have believed in divine healing as a present reality since I was thirty-three years old experiencing firsthand healing after a divorce in a prayer counseling session at a friend's Presbyterian church. Hundreds of people were praying for me. Since I didn't know I had anything except MCI, I still had hope. Had I suspected something different I may have been more despairing.

4
Fingerprints Wiped Away

Hugh

January 2013 ushered in one of the most turbulent years Sharon and I had experienced. She was slipping rapidly into what felt to both of us like a deepening abyss of disability. By the end of the year, she was functioning at nearly normal levels in all aspects of her life. The weeks and months between those extremes are where the turbulence occurred.

I recall a morning in late December 2012, when I was awakened at six-thirty in the morning by Sharon leaning against the bottom of the bed, clinging to the bedpost. "Are you all right?" I asked as I walked around to her.

"I can't stand up," she replied.

"Okay, just hold on." I got behind her. "I've got you. Try to let go." As soon as she did her knees buckled. I worked her around to where she could get back into the bed. She tried to speak, but couldn't form words and quickly fell back asleep.

Three hours later we were in the dining room for breakfast. One of Sharon's morning routines involved using a Spiriva inhaler for her asthma. She would open a foil packet, remove a cylindrical capsule and place it in the inhaler, close the mouthpiece, and inhale deeply. She had done this for so long that it was an automatic procedure, yet this time she couldn't coordinate the task. She looked at me with a helpless expression as she said, "I can't remember how to do it."

A year earlier her psychiatrist had asked me to manage her medications because she was getting them confused. Each week I would organize a dispenser box and at each dosage period I would take out the correct meds and place them in front of her with a cup of water. She would then swallow them.

On this morning, she picked up the pills, popped them into her mouth and began chewing. It took me by surprise.

"Honey, don't chew those," I said with alarm. "Swallow them." I handed her the cup, but she didn't seem to know what to do with it. She looked at me with a pleading expression. I put the cup to her lips and we got through the medication issue that time. I soon learned I would need to instruct her to swallow, pill-by-pill, each time.

That night Sharon's incontinence became a problem for both of us. She had gone to bed at eight o'clock, and I had used a few hours after that for writing (I was working on the draft of my second novel at the time). I went to bed at eleven o'clock and was awakened thirty minutes later when Sharon got up to use the bathroom. To prevent her from falling I had to get up with her. This went on until 4:30 a.m. at forty-five-minute intervals. She finally fell into a sound sleep and I had to awaken her for her thyroid medication at 8:30 a.m., after which she slept again.

I left for a doctor's appointment and when I returned at 11:30 a.m. Sharon was still sleeping soundly. When she awakened, she experienced a mixture of confusion and clarity, which continued all day. Sometimes it would seem like she was trying to assess her own functioning. She would ask me, "What day is it?" I would answer and then she'd ask again. The strange part was that at the same time, she was clear about the month, year, holidays, and so forth.

One morning Sharon was standing in the bathroom brushing her teeth, and I was in the adjoining bedroom. I heard her exclaim something and then there was a "thump." She had fallen against the wall and then slumped to the floor. I dropped what I was doing and rushed to her. "What happened? Are you okay?"

"I don't know how I fell," she said.

"Did you hurt yourself?"

"No," she said quietly.

When I helped her up she was unsteady, listing to the left with a tendency to fall backwards. I helped her get dressed and into her transport chair, and we ate breakfast without further incident. In fact, things went better all day until just after supper. At meal time I would roll her up to the table and then lock the wheels on her chair. That gave me the freedom to finish cooking, serve the meal, eat my own supper and then clean up the kitchen.

We have a round table and she had always sat with her back to the kitchen. On this occasion, everything had gone well through supper. She was at the table while I cleaned the dishes. On impulse, I turned around from the sink and saw her standing up behind her chair, pulling on it.

"What are you doing?" I asked, turning from the sink. Every unexpected movement she made was alarming to me. Often Sharon did things quickly and quietly. She said nothing as she fell backwards into the kitchen, hitting her head against the floor. She seemed frightened and confused but had no visible injuries. I helped her up and for the next hour we watched television. Then she went to bed. Once she was settled, I went across the hall to do some writing in my office. I left the door open and asked her to call me if she needed help. She said she would, then dropped off to sleep.

At ten o'clock I heard the bedroom door open, so I got up to check on her. She was standing unsteadily beside the bed, with a confused expression on her face.

"What time is supper?" she asked.

"Honey, we already ate supper. It's nighttime now."

"When do I take my meds?"

"You've already taken them," I said, helping her back into bed. That seemed to satisfy her and she went to sleep.

The next day she didn't seem as confused, but she fell in the bathroom, and had difficulty walking, a pattern that became the norm throughout the month. The frequency of falls increased. Almost every day there was a time when she didn't know the day, date, time or month. She did always seem to know the year. Every day seemed to bring new challenges and I felt that I had to be right with her at all times.

Sharon's falls brought challenges in getting her back on her feet. We developed a system whereby I would pull her up by extending my arms to her, placing her feet against mine toe-to-toe, and pulling her upright. She would wobble a bit and then her tension would release. Even a simple maneuver like getting her out of the car and then turning her to sit in her transport chair become a challenge, because she would sway as if to fall.

To combat her increasing incontinence, her urologist prescribed a new medication that brought some relief. Dietary guidelines led to reducing sodium, and eating fish and chicken much of the time. With each adjustment Sharon seemed to make progress, but then a new level of need would emerge.

The previous fall her primary care physician had prescribed an Exelon Patch at Sharon's request, in an effort to counter some of her memory loss. By January we had seen no benefit and discontinued using it. At this point, anything that could be taken out of the daily routine was helpful as long as there were no adverse effects.

Self-care is critical and challenging for full-time caregivers, and I had a couple of issues to deal with. For one thing, I was diagnosed with prostate cancer in 2011 and have been in a program of watchful waiting ever since. One critical activity the doctor prescribed was walking, so I developed a pattern of walking two miles around our neighborhood several mornings a week. I continued to do that as long as possible, but there came a time when I knew it was not safe to leave Sharon in the house alone.

I discovered that one morning when I returned from another activity I had maintained for self-care, which was attending a weekly breakfast gathering with a group of pastors, most of whom are retirees. The Wednesday breakfast fellowship became a valuable support group. We developed a routine. I would get Sharon up for her thyroid medication, and then she would go back to sleep while I took my half-hour walk or went to my hour-and-a-half breakfast meeting. I would leave her a message in bold print on a 4x6 note card that I taped to the lamp bedside her bed, so that if she awakened she would know where I was. Week after week I would find her still sleeping soundly when I returned, so we felt this was a safe plan.

On January 16, however, I came back from breakfast and found Sharon lying on the floor in the hall. She appeared confused, almost dazed.

"How did you get on the floor?" I asked.

"I've been scooting around the house," she replied.

Seeing that the desk lamp in her office had been turned on, I concluded that she had gotten up and somehow gone in there. She would always answer me honestly when I asked a direct question, and she told me she had gone into her office to look through a catalog. She didn't remember how she got there. This was a wake-up call for me. I stopped attending the breakfast meetings. I also stopped walking and switched to doing some sciatic nerve exercises in the house.

Such was the pattern throughout January and into the next month. It became impossible to run errands, like going to the grocery or pharmacy, without help. A small, wonderful group of women from Sharon's circle at church volunteered to assist, and we set up two days a week when women would come in to sit with her while I did errands. They also came on Friday afternoons so I could continue attending my Writer's Critique group at the Lifelong Learning Institute in Midlothian, Virginia.

Writing, in fact, became one of my best self-care activities. During these early months of the year I was involved in developmental editing of my first novel. It was an extensive process during which I also began to re-think the structure of my partially written second novel.

Publishing could be done by email, so I would follow guidelines and submit revisions online. Offline I would go back into re-writing my other book. This kept my mind engaged and my efforts focused on something outside the stress of daily caregiving.

In addition to all of this, I prayed constantly about Sharon's condition, and my own coping. One answer came to me repeatedly— "Wait." I sensed in my spirit that healing would come. My key was to live one day at a time, trusting in God's daily provision. All would be well in time.

□□□

Sharon

I don't remember much from either 2012 or the first half of 2013. I do, however, remember being impulsive, getting up out of my chair, forgetting that I fell most times when I stood up. I don't think I could really see myself as being at the level of disability at which I was actually functioning. I was typically a cautious person.

With the tremor getting worse, I couldn't even write my name.

Even though Hugh would tell me where he was going, I often forgot and would become scared when I was alone. My confidence slipped away. All I could do was to sleep while he was gone. All these things are like fingerprints in my mind that have been wiped away.

5
A Glimmer of Hope

Hugh

The Psalmist directs a profound thought toward God when he says, *"I praise you, for I am fearfully and wonderfully made."* (Psalm 139:14 NRSV) When Sharon tells me she can't remember the trauma she experienced during her difficult days of decline, I can understand. What a blessing that God has created our brains with the capacity to wipe away from consciousness those things that, were we to fully recall them, would simply break us apart.

As January rolled into February there were times when Sharon simply could not move her left foot, and when she moved her right foot, she threw herself off balance. Her disabilities increased daily. The simplest things, like feeding herself, became impossible tasks. I had to help her eat when she couldn't remember how to move her fork from her plate to her mouth. She could no longer get in or out of the shower, so we got a shower chair and I helped her bathe and dried her off. I learned to comb and style her hair, and apply her makeup. We made a game out of it. We even found some occasions for laughter amidst the pain.

Incontinence and imbalance were the two greatest problems, and they prevented either of us from getting a good night's sleep. The impact of that was different for Sharon than for me, because she would just doze off during a good portion of each day. I learned to sleep lightly and sporadically, yet stay alert.

I made notes about these instances that I shared with her doctors. We were using Depends briefs. Some nights she would go through as many as eight Depends, sometimes wetting either the bed or floor despite using them. I felt we were rapidly approaching the point where something would have to change—but what?

I don't recall the exact timing now, but at some point early in February I called Chesterfield County, Virginia's Social Services and they sent a social worker and nurse to do an assessment on Sharon. One of their suggestions was that I get certified nursing assistants in so that I didn't break myself down. They gave me a list of agencies and I made a few calls and selected Care Advantage for a consultation. They sent out a nurse and social worker and made suggestions for how we might benefit from their services.

One thing that evolved was renting a hospital bed and a commode chair. The equipment was delivered on a Friday and with the help of the church women who sat with Sharon on Tuesdays and Fridays, we made room for the hospital bed next to the queen size bed, which allowed room to move around, and to pull the commode chair to the bedside when needed. The bed had sides that we raised, and I rigged a bell she could ring if she had a need when I wasn't in the room.

Despite her not remembering the hospital bed now, Sharon was quite aware of it at the time. The height of the queen-sized bed seemed to spur a deep-seated fear within her, probably fed by a subconscious awareness of her falls. She was there when the hospital bed arrived and had a say in how we arranged the room to accommodate it.

This was about the time Sharon switched to using a wheelchair. While I was vacuuming the rug one day she jumped up, then came crashing back down onto the transport chair, stressing it in such a way that it became unusable. At night Sharon seemed to have a sense of security related to where I put the wheelchair when she went to bed. These are the kind of memories her brain has now screened from her.

Once we had the hospital bed I developed a pattern of sleeping with an awareness of every sound Sharon made. The sound of the bed springs would tell me she was trying to get up. Most of the time I could jump out of bed and reach her before she tried to stand up. I bought extra twin-size sheets and pillow cases because some nights her bladder would release before I could reach her. We could go through all those sets of bed linens in a single night.

Most of the time Sharon's conversational responses were vague and task-oriented. She was usually compliant and frequently appreciative toward me and others. One day just before Valentine's Day the phone rang. It was a friend whom we had known since my days as pastor of Belmont Church. He sang with a barbershop quartet called the New Virginians. "Do you and Sharon have plans for Valentine's Day?" he asked. I told him we'd be right there at the house. "Our quartet will be going to a few shut-ins to sing that day, and I wondered if Sharon would like to have us come by your house?"

I told him we would welcome them. They arrived at midday, bearing a bouquet of roses, and a brief repertoire of songs. We invited them into the living room and I could feel both Sharon's surprise, and her appreciation. These men warmed both our hearts. Sharon does recall that occasion today, although she doesn't remember the titles of the songs they sang.

Two other significant things happened in February. I knew we were just biding time until I would have to have certified nursing help on some basis, and we lacked the financial resources to do that. So, I applied for Medicaid. The social worker suggested that we apply for long-term home nursing care, which we did. It was a long process, but by the middle of March, we had qualified and this gave us fresh hope that we could pursue whatever became necessary for her care.

The other thing was the result of a process that had begun in January. For several years I had been raising the question of Normal Pressure Hydrocephalus, and usually it ended up as a possibility, but nothing else seemed to happen. Then I had a phone call from Sharon's younger son, who had seen something about NPH online.

He gave me the website, and I pulled it up. It contained a self-test which Sharon took, answering every question affirmatively. Her score indicated a solid basis for seeking a spinal tap to determine if she had NPH, and a "letter to your doctor" that we could print out and take to her primary care physician.

It seemed that once we had this self-test and letter in hand, new doors opened. She was sent for a CT scan and a battery of tests with the same neuropsychologist she had seen before. The results of the scan didn't show much change, but the psychological tests showed a huge change. As a result, her doctor made a referral to a neurosurgeon. We went to see him on February 25. I still recall the scenario in his office.

"Mrs. Harris, can you walk for me?" he asked.

"I'll try," she said. She was sitting in her transport chair and he helped her get up, then held her hands and observed as she tried to walk toward him. She could barely move her feet, listed to the left, and leaned backwards. She couldn't walk at all, so we helped her back into her chair, and he took us through a series of questions, then examined her verbally. He explained what NPH was and how excessive cerebrospinal fluid was not being absorbed by her brain, causing it to pack into some of her brain cavities. One of the primary symptoms was gait disturbance, along with memory loss, incoherence, and incontinence.

"I think you might have NPH," he said, "but there's a test we need to do to determine that for certain. It's an outpatient surgical procedure where we will insert a tap into the base of your spine. Then we'll place you in the ICU unit where we'll draw a small amount of fluid at specific intervals over a three-day period, and we'll have occupational and physical therapists assess how you respond as the fluid is drawn away from your brain."

The spinal tap was set for March 18, and we went home with a glimmer of hope that things were finally moving forward. In all of this we had prayer support from family, friends and our church, and we shared our joy with all of them. The prayers continued as we prepared to take a new step in March.

□□□

Sharon

To think that I had earned two Master's Degrees and now couldn't remember what day it was felt so upsetting. During the time Hugh is describing, I felt as though an opaque shade had been drawn over my brain. I silently wondered if this was how patients with Alzheimer's Disease felt.

The fact that I cannot remember Christmas of 2012 is unthinkable. Christmas is a season I enjoy tremendously. The music, gift giving, and special church events and services always thrill me. It seems surprising that singing Christmas carols this past year did not resurrect any memories from the year before.

Hugh was wonderful at "normalizing" things. When I read his thoughts now, although I don't remember the events, I realize that he kept me from falling into despair. He has a wonderful sense of humor, so his making a game of things like showering me and styling my hair, are not as painful and traumatic as they might be as reminders of my condition. I believe the fact that he had a brother who was six years younger and profoundly disabled with cerebral palsy sensitized him to my condition. I can't remember more than one or two occasions when he became impatient or exasperated with me.

Still, I have no memory of sleeping in a hospital bed or of using a commode chair. The bed was returned to the rental company when I no longer needed it. There are several assistive devices stored in our garage. When I look at those now I can pull up some memory of having used each one of them. I also have a cane and plastic leg brace that remind me of having been misdiagnosed with drop foot by physical therapists.

The trip to the neurosurgeon's office is another thing I don't remember. I do know that during this time it always felt like my feet were glued to the floor, so it is not surprising that I could not walk steadily for him.

As a former licensed professional counselor, I am aware of research indicating that everything we experience is stored in the brain. The fact that I can't currently access some of my memory from 2009 through July 2013 does not mean that I will never remember those events. I cannot presently remember just how disabled I was, but sometimes glimpses of recollection do occur. For instance, just the mention of a bell on the hospital bed signals something deep within me when I ring that bell now.

I do remember that we applied for Medicaid, but Hugh acted on my behalf through his Power of Attorney (POA). Had I understood that it was for long-term nursing care, I would have been appalled and angry. By God's grace, that detail did not reside in my conscious memory.

6

Detour

Hugh

On Monday afternoon, March 11, 2013, Sharon and I took the first step into a new dimension of her journey as we signed in at the surgical center of a local hospital. The modern, open structure, with its multi-storied glass front, felt inviting as we settled in and browsed through the papers we had been instructed to bring.

Soon her name was called, and we went to an intake cubicle where her basic information was processed and papers signed. Then she was shown to an examining room where she was evaluated in preparation for surgery at 8:00 a.m. on Monday, March 18.

I weighed the state of care Sharon now required, as well as my own growing fatigue from twenty-four-seven caregiving. At this point each night was a marathon of her having to go to the bathroom, and each day a marathon of assistance with everything from bathing and hair washing to eating. Sometimes she would not even recognize me and would ask, "When is Hugh coming back?" I knew it was time to get skilled help

The first Certified Nursing Assistant (CNA) came at 9:00 a.m. on Thursday, March 14, and stayed five hours. She got Sharon up, bathed and dressed her, got breakfast for her, then stayed with her while I took care of errands and work tasks. She left after Sharon went down for her nap at 2:00 p.m. While Sharon slept, I worked on my writing. I got her up when it was time to fix supper, after which we watched Wheel of Fortune and Jeopardy together. I got her back to bed for the night around 8:45 p.m.

On Friday the CNA followed the same procedure, only she stayed until 4:30 p.m. so that I could attend my writer's critique group that afternoon. On Saturday and Sunday she did the five-hour routine again, except that Sunday, the night before Sharon's surgery, I had another CNA come in to sit with her overnight. I slept in another room to be fresh the next day. Sharon seemed to like the people who worked with her, and she was always cooperative.

Monday was THE BIG DAY. At 8:00 a.m. we reported to the hospital surgical center. Sharon was taken to a preparation area and I went to the waiting room where I did some writing and talked to several people who came by to offer prayer and support. Her surgeon had said that if she responded as quickly to the spinal tap as he hoped she would, he could proceed with implanting a ventricular-peritoneal shunt after she spent a day or two in observation. I had great expectation that this is exactly what would happen.

Finally, a call came to the waiting room telling me Sharon was in surgery. She would be moved to a Neurosurgical Intensive Care room as soon as the tap was completed. It seemed like a surprisingly short time until her surgery was completed, and she spent some time in recovery. Finally, I received word that she had been transferred to ICU and I could go visit her.

That was another surprise. In my experience, most Intensive Care rooms have very specific, limited visitation times, even for family. The neurosurgical unit, however, was open most of the time throughout the day. I sat in the room with Sharon while she slept, occasionally arousing for treatments or meals. The technology involved in this neurosurgical environment overwhelmed me, right down to the way the room was organized. The room was large, with her bed placed right in the center. Two control panels, containing all the equipment usually placed against a wall, were mounted from the ceiling beside her bed. It was possible for the nurses and technicians to rotate this equipment around her, according to each specific need or task.

I was editing my first novel at the time and was told that I could remain in her room while I worked on my laptop computer. That first evening I stayed for a while, saw that she was sleeping most of the time, and then went home for the night. I returned each day to work in the room with her, giving me opportunities to relate to her when she was alert. I was also able to observe the procedure as they did periodic spinal taps and tested her reactions. One of the benefits of that arrangement is that I can now tell her things she cannot recall from that time.

After such an intensive time of caregiving, stepping into an empty house the first night after Sharon's surgery felt strange. I had anticipated being able to sleep through the night once I did not have to keep jumping up to care for her. In reality, my body could not make the adjustment as fast as I had anticipated. All night I kept waking up, thinking I should check on her, then realizing that she wasn't there. As I fixed breakfast the first morning of Sharon's ICU time, I could not shake a haunting, disquieting sense that all was not well.

When I arrived at the hospital, however, things were basically the same as when I had left the night before. Sharon was asleep. When she awoke, she seemed foggy. I desperately wanted to see things I could call "progress" in her responses, and I imagined that I did see them. However, she was not responding as expected. Periodically the staff would draw off some spinal fluid and then measure the results. Gait improvement was a major indicator the medical staff sought, but when they got Sharon up she couldn't move her feet and continued to lean to the left and backwards.

Finally, on Thursday, after only slight results had been demonstrated from the spinal tap, her neurosurgeon informed me that she did not meet the criteria for implantation of a shunt in her brain. Because the spinal tap was an outpatient procedure, she could only stay three days for observation and testing.

I remember asking the doctor, "Where does that leave us?"

He explained again about the NPH protocol and said she would need to be in a safe place with round-the-clock care.

"If she doesn't have NPH, then what is her diagnosis?" I asked.

"The only thing I can say at this point is *irreversible dementia*," he said. Next, a social services representative from the hospital went to work seeking a facility where she could be moved. I felt totally devastated. Anger, disappointment, and futility raged within me. I felt totally helpless, and struggled to hang on to the faith and confidence that had propelled my efforts up to this point. Somewhere in the recesses of my spirit I heard God saying, "Patience. Wait. All will be well."

Efforts to find an available bed in a local facility proved to be difficult. For a time, it looked like Sharon would be transferred to Goochland County, to the west of Richmond, about fifty miles from our home. Then that fell through. The next opening was in Farmville, Virginia, which was about seventy miles from our home. I could not imagine visiting her regularly at that distance, and keeping up with everything else. I asked the social worker to keep searching, hoping for something else to surface. We were running out of time.

On Friday, the social worker asked me to help her search by going to some facilities and checking them out while she stayed on the phone. I visited several places, and felt a little more confident as I toured the facilities and saw the nature of care they provided. I put Sharon on some waiting lists, but there were no Medicaid beds available. Finally, I pulled into the parking lot at the hospital, resigned to the seventy-mile trek to Farmville, when my cell phone rang.

"I'm calling for Hugh Harris," the voice on the phone said. "We have a bed that has just become available for your wife." Tears of joy burst forth as I hung up, said a prayer of thanksgiving, and rushed in to find the social worker to get the transfer process moving. I didn't know much about Hopewell, but I did know it was much closer to our home. I knew that somehow God had worked this out. He was not finished with Sharon yet.

I checked Sharon out of the hospital as evening shadows began to form, and we struck out for the town of Hopewell, where she was being transferred. We stopped to eat a quick supper in the car at a local restaurant, then drove on, arriving after seven o'clock that evening. The facility had easy access from the interstate highway, and we soon pulled to the entrance of a two-story brick building with an arched canopy.

The staff had been expecting us. Someone was waiting at the office when we entered. Sharon was assigned to a room and I gave her portfolio to the supervising nurse, then helped her get settled. Finally, I said goodnight and drove 23 miles home.

As I prayed that night, I had an overwhelming sense of relief. I felt challenged to trust God and avoid getting hooked into the outcome *I* wanted to see. I poured out my soul and tried to bargain with God in my grief.

"She's too young for this," I yelled. "It's too soon. She has so much to give."

My tears flowed and finally in exhaustion I could hear that small inner voice again. "It's okay. Wait. All will be well." My tension eased and I went to bed sensing that Sharon was simply on a temporary detour along the road to full recovery. She *did* have NPH. I *knew* it. God was in this and somehow, we would get back on track.

□□□

Sharon

The only memory I have is going with Hugh to the hospital for the pre-admission review. It seemed very early to me (although I believe it was 12:30 p.m.) and it seemed to take forever, since I did have complete recall of my medical history. I do not recall being in the ICU unit, receiving periodic spinal taps, or being asked to walk and perform other tasks to measure my progress.

I remember nothing until I was recovering from the surgery. Hugh tells me he waited for me in the neurosurgical unit's waiting room. I remember trying to put sentences together to converse intelligently with the recovery room nurses. I remember that I felt embarrassed and asked them to forgive me.

7

Back on Track

Hugh

Sharon's first weekend at the health care center went smoothly. On Saturday, I couldn't tell how well she understood her situation. I was surprised how settled she seemed. The staff was skilled and responsive to her needs. They were aware of the danger of falls and had assigned her a wheelchair and activated alarms on that and her bed to prevent her from getting up without someone knowing about it. The staff members I talked to were pleasant and knowledgeable about the people in their care.

Sharon's roommate suffered from Multiple Sclerosis. She was bedridden except when lifted hydraulically and transferred to a wheelchair. She also had speech complications. She had a television set that she kept on above her bed, and she got all sorts of intellectual stimulation from PBS and other programs. Sharon's deep sensitivity came through as she related to her and they quickly formed a bond.

On Sunday morning I went with Sharon to a worship service led by a local pastor in the dining room. I was amazed how many residents attended. The service was spirited, and marked by the pastor's sensitivity to the people he served. He had someone with him who led praise singing, after which he went among the people, inviting them to share their testimonies. Next, he read the scripture, offered a prayer, then preached a message of hope and encouragement. I soon learned that this and other services, plus Bible studies each week, served as spiritual anchors for residents.

The facility had a policy permitting family members to purchase a meal ticket and eat with residents. I was able to stay after worship and eat with Sharon in the dining room. Most Sundays I attended the early service at our church and then went to the care facility for Sharon's service, followed by lunch. Sometimes we played Scrabble when the conference room two doors down from her room was available, or went outside to a gazebo beside a small pond to watch the Canadian geese come and go.

On Tuesday morning after Sharon was admitted, I attended a meeting about her care. There were seven staff members present representing everything from administration to housekeeping. We went over her contract for care which I then signed. Food service talked about their services, and we talked about medications and other health issues. Most memorable to me were the people from Occupational, Physical and Speech Therapy, who shared an elaborate set of goals they intended to accomplish with Sharon.

I remember sitting there wondering: *do they really know her? Are we talking about the same person?* When they finished their presentation, I felt I had to speak.

"You do know, of course, that Sharon's diagnosis is *irreversible dementia*. I love the sound of all that you've outlined here, but it doesn't sound like where she is. Do you really think these goals are practical?"

"Absolutely," came the answer. "We know her diagnosis, but we also know the capacity of people to respond when given the right stimulus and motivation. We may not achieve all of these goals, but our job is to take her as far as she can go."

I left there impressed with two things. First, this was not just an institutional facility, but a *family* of caring, connected people. They knew their residents and cared about each one. Second, there was obviously a spiritual quality at the heart of the operation. I remember so many times after that when I thanked God for having sent us to this place. My faith in Sharon's healing was reinforced.

As it turned out, the therapy staff was effective in their work. They scheduled Sharon for regular sessions throughout the day. Sometimes I sat in on those when I went to visit. Sharon was open and receptive, and tried hard to do what was asked of her. Gradually her functioning improved.

One of Sharon's key symptoms had been incontinence, and she tended to try going to the bathroom on her own whenever the urge moved her. A change in that behavior was one of the first indications she was making progress. So was her ability to move her feet, and her memory was improving. Within a few weeks she was walking down the hall with a walker, and she was proud to announce her progress each time I visited her.

We had a surgical follow-up appointment scheduled with the neurosurgeon on April 10. By that time Sharon had shown so much improvement that the doctor seemed surprised, given her condition three weeks earlier after the spinal tap. He had her stand from a seated position. She was able to walk, although haltingly and with some list to the side and backwards, but she was obviously doing much better at this primary task. Short-term memory was improving, and we had now gotten a better handle on her incontinence, as well as some reduction in her tremor.

"This is what we wanted to see after the spinal tap," the doctor told her. "If this continues, I would say a VP Shunt is not out of the picture. Come back in a month and we'll see how you're doing."

We went back to the health care center elated at the prospect. On the following Sunday, I took Sharon to see her new granddaughter, who was born in a different hospital from the one where Sharon had her spinal tap, on the same day the tap had been done. "Grandma" had never seen the baby. Sharon's younger son and his wife live in Chesterfield County about twelve miles from our home. The visit was delightful. Sharon held the baby while I took pictures.

Family support is all important in anyone's recovery from illness. Sharon's other son and his girlfriend visited and attended worship several times. Once we all went out to lunch at a nearby restaurant, which enabled them to experience Sharon's changes first hand, rather than just through phone calls or from what I told them. These connective steps were essential in bolstering a supportive family context for Sharon's healing.

Sharon also had a chance for a day trip to visit her first cousin and her husband in a community outside the Richmond area. She and her cousin share a very close relationship. The last time they had been together had been in February. Now they were amazed at the progress Sharon had made, which was encouraging to us.

By the end of May we were convinced that things were back on track. The surgery to implant the VP shunt was scheduled and we anticipated a dramatic return to normalcy.

ㅁㅁㅁ

Sharon

After moving from the hospital to the healthcare center, I felt glad to be settled again. I slept well except for the usual two times I awakened to go to the bathroom that was attached to my room. How small and drab that bathroom was. I believe I was wearing adult diapers by this time in the progression of NPH. Incontinence was a major insult since I was only 65 years old.

My roommate was a woman near my age. I learned much more than I had ever known about Multiple Sclerosis from her. We could, with much effort on my part, communicate. She had once designed a home and lived in it, enjoyed classical music, and kept up with world events through her television. Her food had to be pureed due to the effects of her condition, but when I left she was doing better, thanks to physical therapy, I believe.

Going to a church service on the premises of the healthcare center normalized life for me. Hugh was always there to roll me down to the dining hall in my wheelchair. It became a special hour during the week. So was the fine lunch prepared and served by the kitchen staff. Especially wonderful were the times my older son and his girlfriend came for lunch. I had a lot to catch up on.

I felt myself getting stronger, even though I sometimes struggled from working so diligently in PT, OT and speech therapy.

8

Over the Top

Hugh

The pre-admission routine on May 28 was a repeat of what we had done before the spinal tap. Our schedule for the VP shunt was confirmed for Tuesday, June 4 at 7:30 a.m. This time it would be an inpatient procedure with admission following surgery. To arrive at the hospital two hours ahead of surgery, we had to leave the healthcare center by 4:45 a.m. That took a lot of coordination, but everyone pitched in, and we made it on time—only to find out once we had reached the hospital that surgery had been rescheduled for later in the day.

Everything seemed to click in place, however, and after the shunt was implanted Sharon was sent to the rehabilitation floor from the recovery room. This was an entirely different scenario from her experience in the neurological ICU in March. She was still a little fuzzy about things that evening, but I could see improvement in her functioning by the next day. She shared a semi-private room with a woman who had had a knee replacement revision. Each of them had rehab scheduled at various times throughout the day. Sharon was very positive, and after ten days in the hospital, she was ready for her remaining twenty days of inpatient care in another facility. We had to choose someplace to go.

"Why not see if the same healthcare center you were in has a room for you?" I asked. "After all, it's because of their quality of care that you're here now."

"I agree," Sharon said, and I called to see if this was possible to get her back in. The staff was once again able to accommodate her needs. She went back knowing this time that it was for a limited stay. No more long-term care issues. No more incontinence. No more danger of falling. No more wheelchair. They assigned her a walker, and she began to walk the halls when accompanied by me or a therapist. The therapy staff worked with her on a wide range of issues aimed toward returning her to a normal life at home without assistive equipment.

Ten months after Sharon's release to return home, we went back to the healthcare center for a visit. Sharon has had trouble remembering everything about the facility. We wondered if going back to experience the setting and talking to staff members would trigger some memories. The greeting we received was overwhelming.

"Sharon, is that you?"

"Look at you. I can't believe it."

"It's so good to see you doing so well. We're so glad you came to visit."

These were some of the many expressions we heard as we went in on that Sunday afternoon. We visited Sharon's former roommate, taking her a gift of her favorite body wash, and walked into the conference room where we had sometimes played Scrabble. We walked the halls, looked into the shower room, went out to the gazebo to see the Canadian Geese, and visited the rehabilitation center and activity rooms.

Most of the staff members Sharon had known were still there. The atmosphere reminded us what a special, caring place this healthcare center is. The therapist on duty texted Sharon's speech therapist, who was off duty. She made a special effort to come in and see Sharon. It was a great reunion. Visiting there again, I recalled the hopefulness I always felt when I came in the door.

After Sharon's inpatient postsurgical rehab, she still needed some help. We were qualified for another thirty days of in-home physical and occupational therapy, so I called the agency I had used earlier. They sent two wonderful women to work with us.

Somehow I had thought that when the CSF was drained from the brain, there would be an almost instant return to normal functioning. It didn't quite work like that. There were many areas of quick recovery, but in other areas time and assistance was still needed. That's what the in-home care was about.

The occupational therapist came to our home three days in July. She helped Sharon with sequencing, so that she could remember how to cook again. The physical therapist came eight days in July and one in August. By the time these dedicated people had completed their work, Sharon was ready to take a vacation—something I had wondered, just a few months earlier, if we would ever experience again.

After the brief vacation, we devised a plan for Sharon to get walking exercise. A key activity for me over recent years has been doing a two-mile fitness walk in our neighborhood several days a week. In the past, Sharon and I had walked the corridors at Chesterfield Towne Center, a local shopping mall, once each week. That old experience came back into my mind.

"Do you remember how we used to walk in the mall?" I asked.

"Yes, I do. I also remember that it got to be too much for me at some point and we stopped doing it."

"Well, maybe that was an early part of the spinal fluid buildup. Maybe your decline was going on a lot longer than we thought. But I have been thinking—at the healthcare center you walked the halls, which is very much like walking in the mall. I'll bet we could go there a couple of mornings a week and do some very limited walking. What do you think?"

"If there's a place to sit down, that might work. I can't walk very far without resting."

I knew that in the older section of the mall the hallways were shorter, and had seen chairs placed in the center of that area, and at the end of each corridor. I told her about that and said, "Let's try it, okay?"

"Okay," she said, and we began the experiment. Sharon was walking very slowly now, and still listing somewhat to the side, but not leaning backwards. We would walk from one set of chairs to the next, rest, then do another section. She could walk about thirty feet at a time. Gradually, her stamina improved, and her walking stabilized. We found that we needed to be intentional about efforts to bring back her normal functioning. Progress was slow, for sure, but we were cresting the top of the hill, beginning to accelerate the journey toward the finish line of full functioning.

□□□

Sharon

While I do remember getting up early to go to the hospital for the shunt implantation, I don't remember the rescheduling. I recall the surgeon introducing me to two staff members who would assist him. As I recall, both were young (probably under thirty). I don't recall meeting the anesthesiologist, but I'm sure I did. The lights in the operating room were very large and bright. Soon I was put under anesthesia.

Next came the worst of the post-op time. What I remember is the horrible agitation I felt and verbalized, which I believe was an adverse reaction to being given morphine. Nurses in the small room in which I went through this harrowing experience were patient and vigilant. I do remember asking them to forgive me for my rant.

Back in my room, I was thankful to have good friends as visitors with whom I could converse reasonably well. I'm thankful for all who came.

I frequently felt the space on my head that had been shaved. The covering for the two-and-a-quarter-inch valve felt like papier mache. The stitches were removed after several days. Now I can only feel the valve for the VP shunt and the raised skin for the two catheters that drain the excess CSF. My neurosurgeon told me there would be five holes in my head for the shunt insertion. Even my hair stylist was a part of my support system. He styled my hair attractively as it was growing out.

The hospital rehabilitation team was wonderful. I bounced a large ball, threw a small ball, walked up three steps, and back down again. I took every task very seriously. When I qualified for more postsurgical rehab, I was excited. I still do some of the prescribed exercises, and am back to cooking a little again.

Months after all the outpatient rehabilitation therapy was over, Hugh and I visited the healthcare center once again, as he has said. I remembered the names of most of the staff that was working that Sunday afternoon. I was really glad to revisit and to thank all who had helped me regain my health and normal functioning.

Though my former roommate was lying flat in bed, rather than sitting in a wheelchair after gall bladder surgery, she told me she could finally have an afternoon snack that wasn't pureed, thanks to her therapist's work. I was thrilled for her. What a persevering spirit she always exhibited, which inspired me.

9
No Turning Back

Hugh

O n August 26 Sharon and I pulled up at one of our favorite hotels in Kill Devil Hills on the North Carolina Outer Banks. This was where we had spent a couple of days in the off season many years ago when we were first married. It had been cold then, and the beach, restaurants and shops had been sparsely occupied. Now we were arriving in the heat of summer and everything was crowded. As we drove toward Nags Head on the Beach Road I took in the growth since our last trip there.

During one of our pastorates, a church family had offered us the use of their beach house in the Jockey's Ridge area of Nags Head. We had spent some wonderfully relaxing times there over the years, until access to the cottage changed. After that we went occasionally, usually staying at a hotel. Our last visit had been with friends in March 2010.

On this trip, we drove on the Beach Road, sand dunes piled high on our left, occasionally catching a glimpse of the breaking surf. There were brightly colored buildings, and shops with kayaks, surf boards and beachwear strung out along the road or on porches. Bicyclists competed with joggers, cars, and families traversing the road from the beach to their cottages. We felt blessed to once again enjoy this place. Only a few months earlier it had seemed to me that such things would only be memories etched in my mind.

"Let's keep a lookout for our hotel," I said. "There seem to be more hotels here now, and I'm having trouble recognizing things."

We rode along, commenting to each other as the things we saw touched our shared memories.

"There it is," Sharon said. "Just past the next traffic light."

"You're right. Thanks for spotting it." We pulled into the parking lot, checked in and went to the room we had reserved earlier on the Internet. "Do you remember the first time we stayed here?" I asked.

"Yes." Now our room faced the parking lot, but the one on our first visit had faced the ocean.

"Remember how we cracked the balcony door open just enough to hear the sound of the surf all night long?"

"I'll never forget it," Sharon said. "The sound of the surf and gulls has always had a tranquil effect on me."

We ate supper in the hotel restaurant, then went out to the deck the hotel had built onto the dunes. We spent some time relaxing in hammock-like chairs, watching the surf and people on the beach. The next two days became special. We went to the beach, visited seafood restaurants, and drove around the village of Manteo. We talked about the charter boat on which we'd taken her now-grown boys fishing (and caught nothing, Sharon remembered) years earlier.

Climbing over the dunes and walking on the beach required all the energy Sharon could muster, but the blessing was that she could do it. She might have been slow, but she was persistent in her efforts. Visiting outlet shops at Corolla put her walking to the acid test, which she passed. As we drove across the causeway to the mainland on our way home, we remarked about the miracles God had performed in her return from dementia.

It had been a brief vacation, but one of the best ever.

Healing from something like NPH is miraculous, but not instant. We were reminded of that on September 7 when Sharon's incontinence and balance issues suddenly resurfaced. This continued on Sunday and Monday, so on September 12 we saw her urologist, who changed her medication. That produced some results, but because gait issues were involved we knew we had to see her neurosurgeon.

We got an appointment with the neurosurgeon on September 23. "Let me see you walk," he said. Sharon walked toward him. After interviewing her and testing her responses, the doctor placed a magnetic instrument over the shunt on her head. It was connected to his computer and he read the data from the shunt.

"There's no problem with the drainage, and that's good," he pronounced. "The shunt is draining the fluid as it should. We want to be careful not to take away too much CSF too quickly and cause a worse problem with water on the brain. I'm going to make an adjustment that I think will relieve the problem, and I'll have you check back in three months." The adjustment worked.

As I have mentioned, one of my coping strategies as a caregiver had been to continue writing my first novel, which I completed by the end of the summer of 2012. I had acquired a publisher, and during the first two months of 2013, I had been involved in a developmental editing process. It was all done digitally, via email.

Remarkably, I had gone through some of the most trying times involving Sharon's spinal tap, with a publisher's deadline right on top of me. During that time, I succeeded in cutting over 40,000 words from my manuscript. This resulted in a tight story that could be offered at a reasonable price. Publishing went forward with a release date of October 15, 2013.

When the first pre-release books were shipped to me in August, I embraced a new challenge of learning how to market my book. It was necessary to sell myself as an author, and then sell my book as a good read with a worthwhile message. This involved book talks and book signings in as many venues as possible. Editing had co-existed with the challenges of caregiving. Now marketing would have to co-exist with the challenges of Sharon's unfolding return to normalcy.

She went with me to some of the book signings, which became a valuable time of bonding for us. I remember our first book signing at a branch of the Chesterfield County Libraries. Sharon went with me then and on several other occasions. Then she became content to stay home by herself while I did some others. Each time we did a library signing I contributed to the Friends of the Library organization, and Sharon joined that group. This became another doorway for her, back out of dementia to normal functioning.

As I have mentioned earlier, during her spinal tap in March Sharon had missed the birth of her newest grandchild, whose baptism we were able to attend on October 13. Even things that are usually considered special, yet taken in stride as an ordinary part of life, become so much more significant when you've been cognitively absent and now have returned enough to participate in those things.

October was the month when Sharon awoke one morning and she was simply "herself" again. Her thinking was clearer, her energy was better, and she seemed more in control of things. We still shared the cooking, and I was still managing her medications, but it began to be more of a shared experience than one where I managed everything.

Piece by piece, Sharon's cognitive functioning seemed to "click" into place.

One of those "clicks" was her memory of a time several years earlier when she had participated in a nutritional weight management and exercise program that had resulted in losing twenty-five pounds, contributing greater balance to her life. When she saw an ad for a new location of this program near us in Chesterfield County, she went for an interview and signed up for another ten-week course. She continued with that program through May 2014, then took a break to do a water aerobics class for seniors at a different facility.

With October's early twinges of changing leaves, and hints of fall in the morning temperatures, it was clear that there was now no turning back for Sharon's full recovery. It would take time, and require patience and effort, but we were firmly on the road.

□□□

Sharon

Relating to grandchildren has always been one of the joys of my life. Hugh had baptized two of our nine grandchildren, and the fact that I could now attend my newest granddaughter's baptism was especially thrilling. Our families gathered for a memorable celebration after the service.

One of the places I really liked for relaxed vacationing was Nags Head, North Carolina. For years, I collected seashells, shopped, and soaked in the sun on this beach. Since I was a baby, pictured in my mother's arms on a visit to my great aunt's home in Norfolk, Virginia in 1948, I had loved the beach, a lake, a pool, a bathtub— any place where there was water. How I had missed our vacations at the beach. Our last vacation had been a trip to the Grand Canyon in 2008. Then we went to Nags Head with a pair of couple friends in March of 2010. I turned down walking with the other two women, fearing I'd have to stop and rest. I was able, nonetheless, to nap and enjoy the fine meals and time we shared.

I was discharged from the healthcare center on July 5, 2013. What a sense of being "reborn." At the same time, I wasn't prepared to be as weak as I found that I was. I had underestimated the fatigue I would feel after returning home. It's easy to forget that after a major surgery there is no bounding back.

I decided to restart a ten-week exercise and weight management program I had done in 2009. I enrolled in the October 31, 2013 class, then did five more months of continuation. By March 31, 2014, I had lost 36 pounds.

I attended every lecture on healthy, nutritious eating and cooking that was offered. I took the free grocery shopping trip and quizzed the fantastic trainers. I was doing two miles in 45 minutes on the Nu-Step machine, along with 45 minutes of weight lifting for balance and strength training. I can optimistically support this program. All the staff deserve kudos.

Now I am again making lifestyle changes. A note here—it feels so freeing to sleep in the bed with my husband, not in a hospital bed with rails up. Turning over and feeling his warm body is something I certainly had missed. I have been eating healthier than ever before, appreciating family and friends, enjoying my return to normalcy, and thanking God for his mercy.

At the same time, I am aware that every day is a gift and that I may need a surgical revision for my shunt in five to seven years. I have been through an incredible journey, and there is no turning back I pray that others will find the kind of help I have received, and for the furtherance of research on NPH. Thanks be to God who gives us victory through the avenues of faith and perseverance.

Sharon's Postscript

I t is now early September 2014. We have just returned from a trip that would have been unthinkable a year-and-a-half ago. At the invitation of a lifelong friend, Hugh and I spent a week in Hilton Head, South Carolina. How refreshing to enjoy a pristine beach at Dolphin Head, on the north side of the island. How inspiring to revel in the fading reddish-gold tones of an inspiring sunset from the deck of a small boat. How relaxing to enjoy a Low Country boiled seafood feast that capped our visit. Over the past year we have both experienced a return to life in dimensions of fullness we will never again take for granted.

We travelled by railroad from Richmond to Savannah to begin our vacation trip. As we checked our bags and validated our e-tickets, we were told our train would be delayed an hour due to problems farther up the line. Hugh made an observation, "Remember how few people there were at this station a few years ago when we traveled to Florida? Look at it now."

The station was alive with activity. We counted at least fifty people waiting within the building as well as outside under blue and white umbrellas. There were people of all ages. The coffee and snack stand was doing a constant business. Gradually different trains arrived and some people left the station to board, while others who detrained picked up their baggage and met friends or family who awaited them. he activity level felt invigorating.

This experience seemed to parallel what has been happening in our lives since my neurosurgery. Like that busy railroad station, our lives have become filled with interests and activities. We have tried to capsulize all of this.

- I continued my fitness program through May, then switched to a weekly hydrolyte water-aerobic program. These activities have enabled me to lose weight and gain stamina and strength. I believe they were invaluable in recovering from the effects of NPH.

- Programs and classes offered by the Chesterfield County Lifelong Learning Institute (LLI) have facilitated my return from dementia. Basic computer courses helped me uncover skills I had either lost, or never could acquire, due to cognitive impairment. During the summer Hugh and I tried a new shared activity through the LLI Reader's Theater class.

- Dementia involves isolation for both the patient and caregivers, so a key to recovery has been intentionally avoiding isolation. The LLI programs have been part of that effort. Another part came as we signed up with a group of Hugh's peers and spouses to attend ten Richmond Squirrels baseball games. Being part of the Silver Squirrels became a healthy addition to our summer schedule.

- Spiritual growth has also been essential for both of us. When Hugh filled in at churches as a retired pastor, he and I were unable to get involved with any depth in our own local church. Then, when he was no longer serving as a pastor, my health issues curtailed our involvement. As 2014 began, however, Hugh took a new step in his life by joining the choir at Providence United Methodist Church where we belong. That has involved commitments to weekly rehearsals and periodic music workshops. In January, we both decided to join a Sunday school class. I have also attended two retreats that have reinforced the spiritual aspects of my total recovery.

- My recovery has also enabled Hugh to invest energy in marketing his books, as well as working on his third novel. I have invested time in researching the medical records from my NPH experience, which has helped in preparing this book. Writing has given us each a healthy perspective on what we've been through, as well as where we want to go with our lives. In addition, Hugh has been involved all summer in doing a series of graphite illustrations of a tourist book being written by a local author and friend.

- Something new in my life last spring was becoming part of the Friends of the Chesterfield County Library, sharing in the opening celebration of the Bon Air Branch following major renovations. Working with the committee and helping with the opening celebration gave me a boost of self-esteem. To think that a year earlier I could not read and comprehend much of anything. Books and libraries have always been important in my life.

My purpose in writing has been to give hope and encouragement to persons who find themselves facing challenges like what Hugh and I have known in recent years. To recap, Normal Pressure Hydrocephalus (NPH) involves the overproduction of Cerebral Spinal Fluid (CSF), which is not adequately absorbed by the brain, resulting in enlarged ventricles and cognitive impairment.

The three major symptoms of NPH are loss of balance and gait, loss of short-term memory, and urinary incontinence. The condition can easily be confused with Alzheimer's Disease (AD), or Parkinson's Disease (PD). If you are experiencing these symptoms, consult with your primary care physician. Tests like a CT Scan or MRI cannot verify NPH in themselves, but they can indicate whether enlarged ventricles exist. In my case, neuropsychological tests also helped define my level of difficulty.

Consult with your doctor about these symptoms. If tests support ventricular enlargement, request consultation with a neurosurgeon. This specialist can order a spinal tap, which measures the change in symptoms as CSF is systematically withdrawn over a test period. This is the definitive test for NPH.

Your neurosurgeon can determine if you would benefit from implantation of a ventriculoperitoneal (VP) shunt, that can be programmed to systematically withdraw CSF, allowing normal functioning to return. An excellent resource for understanding NPH and treatment alternatives is NPH Normal Pressure Hydrocephalus, From Diagnosis to Treatment, by Adam S. Mednick, M.D., Ph.D. (Addicus Books, Omaha, Nebraska, 2013).

If you are a caregiver for someone with symptoms we have described in this book, you have the opportunity to become a patient advocate. By becoming informed, and then advocating for consideration of NPH with doctors, you may be instrumental in opening doors to treatment that might otherwise be overlooked. This is because, according to Dr. Mednick, the incidence of NPH is approximately 5% among all persons who suffer from dementia. Obviously, this presents a very small blip on the diagnostic radar scope, so patient advocacy can help flag the possibility of NPH.

Once a shunt has been implanted, it becomes natural to expect immediate, dramatic improvement. In reality, the effects of NPH may take time to develop, and it is reasonable to allow time for the results of the reduced CSF pressure to show up. My system seems to respond more slowly, but the response does come.

Hugh and I have both learned to walk through recovery with hope and faith, allowing things to unfold as they will. As he has said numerous times, he would pray about my condition, and receive an answer that was often hard to embrace. "Wait. All will be well." Healing has come through the process of waiting with trust.

Hugh and I believe that God is present with us in both our suffering and our healing. At the darkest moments we find God greater than anything we experience, and that gives us hope.

As I conclude, the words of the Twenty-third Psalm come to mind: *"Even though I walk through the valley of the shadow of death, I fear no evil; for thou art with me; thy rod and thy staff, they comfort me."* (Ps. 23:4 RSV).

Sharon French Harris with Hugh Harris

Resources

- Guardian of Hydrocephalus Research Foundation, 2618 Avenue Z, Brooklyn, NY 11235

- Hydrocephalus Association, 4340 East West Highway, Suite 905, Bethesda, MD 29814 Website: www.hydroassoc.org

- Mednick, Adam S. NPH Normal Pressure Hydrocephalus, From Diagnosis to Treatment. Addicus Books, Omaha, Nebraska

NPH Journey into Dementia and Out Again

73958070R00061

Made in the USA
Columbia, SC
08 September 2019